Cover Graphic Designer: Nikki Shavon
Printed in the United States of America
ISBN: 978-1-958117-12-5
Library of Congress Control Number: 2023904038

Publisher: JATNE Publishing, LLC

Table of Contents

INTRODUCTION

The nursing life was a fantastic time filled with learning, growth and getting fully launched into some very adult matters at the young age of 18.

We, the student nurses and young staff nurses, were faced with serious life and death realities on a regular basis.

This memoir is based in the 1980's and shares clips from memories of times past, in my early nursing years. Actually, in a time and place that now seems far removed in many ways from current day practice. Yet, the characters still stand out so many years later. Even the names of some of the patients and staff I still recall. Many of which bring tears to my eyes.

Within this book are glimpses back in time that brings a smile and even laughter. Looking and thinking about nurses of today and how things are done, much may seem prehistoric from my time in the UK.

The nurses world was a fast paced, everchanging work space, where no 2 days were the same. Sometimes it was the best of times and other days it was the worst of times. Fatigue, overwhelm, ranking, rules and hierarchy both spoken and unspoken, modes of conduct and rules of engagement added to the twists and turns of everyday nursing life.

To the reader I trust you will enjoy the memories shared. To my fellow nurses whether past or present, I salute you for the incredible work you have done and continue to put your heart and soul into this amazing work.

Variance in Language

The US and the UK have similar words with a variance in spelling. You will notice some of these italicized in the book. A few are below.

Oedema/Edema

Paediatrics/Pediatrics

Anaesthesia/Anesthesia

There are still some words that require a pause as I consider which side of the Atlantic I'm on and use the correct word or phrase.
(Some words are spelt)
Colour/color
Theatre/theater centre/
center

Traditions

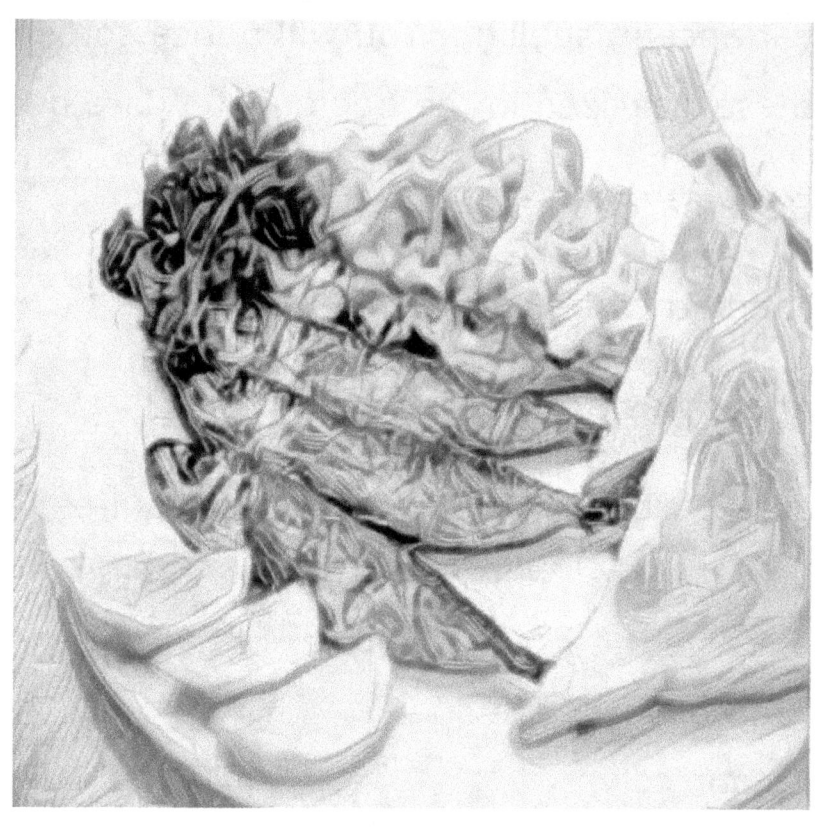

Smoked herring (commonly known as 'Kippers') for breakfast is and was a common delicacy, served on ceramic hospital issue plate and covered with stainless steel plate covers. Quite the pungent scent from this fish, you would always know when it was being served. (I might add it is one of my favorite things at breakfast when in the UK, served with eggs, an amazing fusion of *flavour* from this very salty fish.

Cooked breakfast were still being served on my arrival in the US and does depend on the health care facility. Sometimes traditional and sometimes prepackaged meals. I must admit I was a little perplexed when I saw the prepackaged meal in a plastic tray for the 1st time, all wrapped up rather like the meals that would have been served on international flights.

Formalities

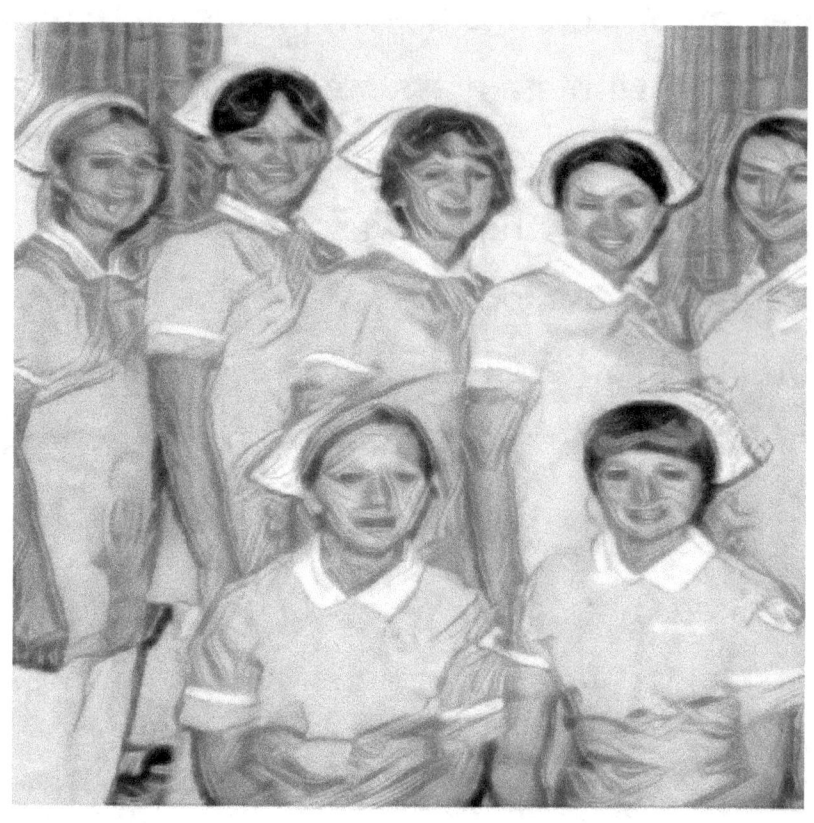

As nurses we were to address each other while on duty and certainly within earshot of a more senior ranking nurse by our last name and adding the word 'nurse' first.

Stateside, it was markedly more casual which seemed initially a bit shocking and strange and at the same time much more relaxed. My manager introduced herself by her 1st name. Dr.'s were addressed by their full title.

Pride

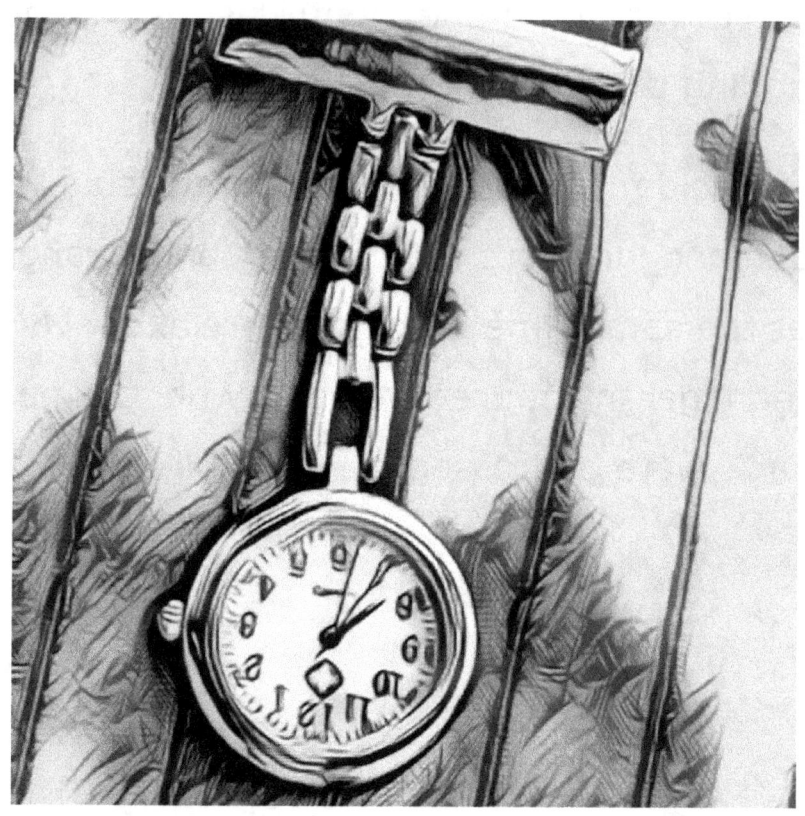

The head nurse if female was known as 'Sister' if male, called 'Charge Nurse'. There wasn't a religious affiliation, just a title. They were mostly female and had a specific uniform which consisted of a cloth nurses cap. There were various styles, but it would be white and more elaborate, even ornate in design, frilly detailing. A white cotton cuff that would go over the ends of the short-sleeved dress to cover the hem of the sleeve. She would be wearing a tightly woven fabric which had very little give and would be worn and secured with an ornately designed silver buckle that met in the front and *centre* which is interlocked to secure it. The students nurse paper cap had a light blue stripe which indicated what year of training she was in. She wore a belt made from the same fabric belt as the student nurses dress uniform. Stateside the head nurse/charge nurse didn't have a particular uniform from everyone else.

Hospitals I worked in had either scrubs with color and design of choice or assigned colours for different staff members, based on their job description, an RN or a nursing assistant. The manager was not typically uniformed but typically had a white lab coat on over street clothes which would indicate medical/nursing staff.

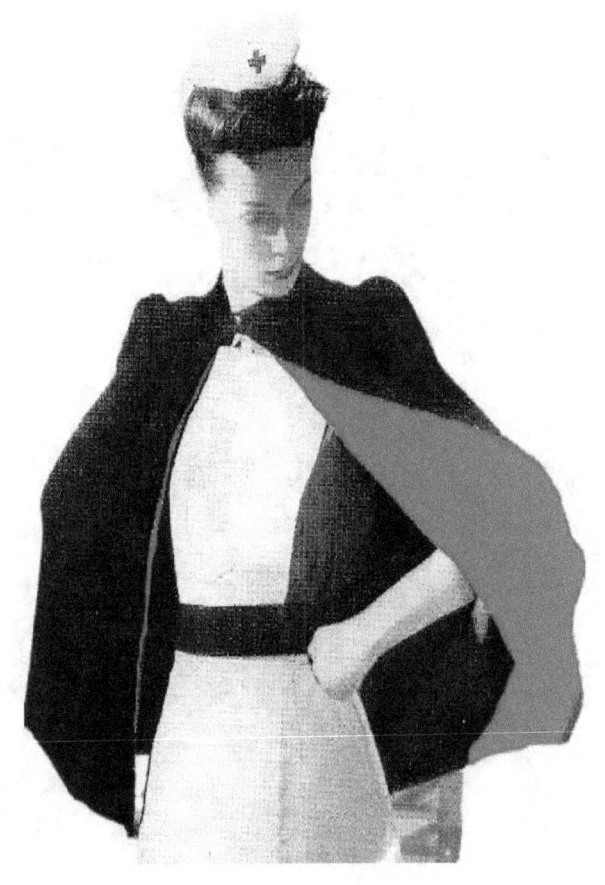

The Qualified Nurse

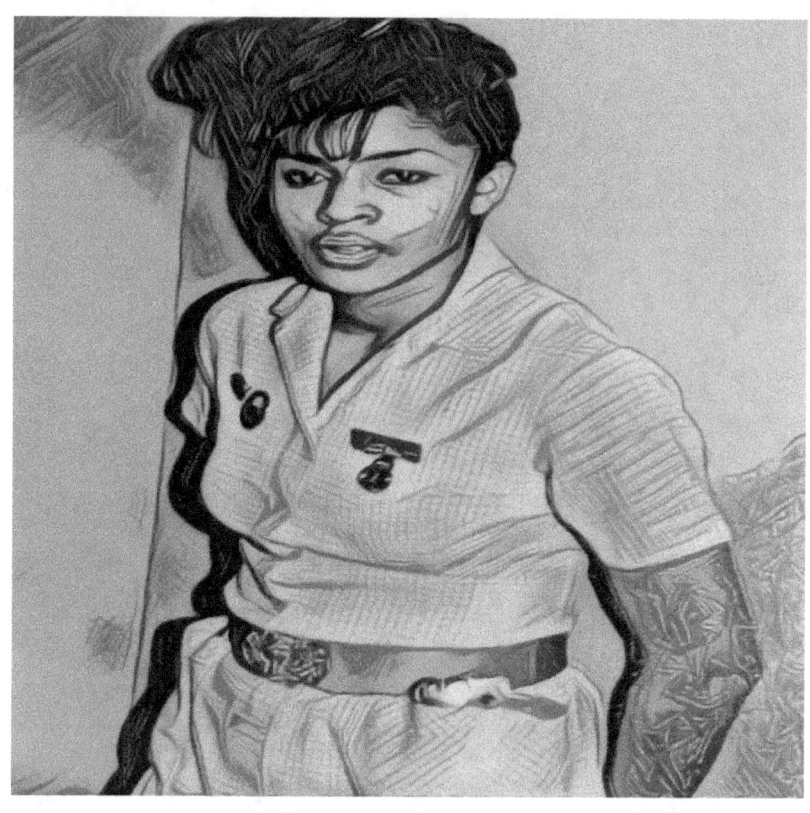

I still have my belt and silver buckle that I chose and purchased from a *jewellery* shop after qualifying as a registered nurse. A light blue belt would indicate the staff nurse's status.

The day of the official announcement to the final year nurses was whether we had passed the Royal College of Nursing exams. There was naturally much buzz amongst us student nurses.

The list of those who had passed the exam was publicized before we received personal letters by mail. Everyone in my class, of about 30, passed the exam. We were all now 'State Registered Nurses ' (SRN). It was a relief to see my name on the list of graduates on the notice board where many had gathered, waiting to peek at the list of those that had passed.

There were relatively new staff nurses in this huddle keen to see the' passed' by the name of fellow nurses they had worked with. It was a proud moment for us, with congratulations and some giggles of relief, the wondering and wait over.

Now onto finding jobs, typically at the hospital that trained us, in-house recruiting. If you got along particularly well with a ward sister and made a great impression during your training, there was often a position already offered when you became a qualified nurse.

My 1st position after qualifying was the exact opposite of my preference!! I would have chosen to work the day shift on a surgical unit (post-surgery patients). Instead, I secured a night shift position on a medical team (Conditions not treated with surgery).

Although we were not all placed in our desired units or *speciality* of choice, we all found positions. Balancing adequate rest and a social life proved to be challenging for me, as the night shift took a toll on my life.

The Nightingale

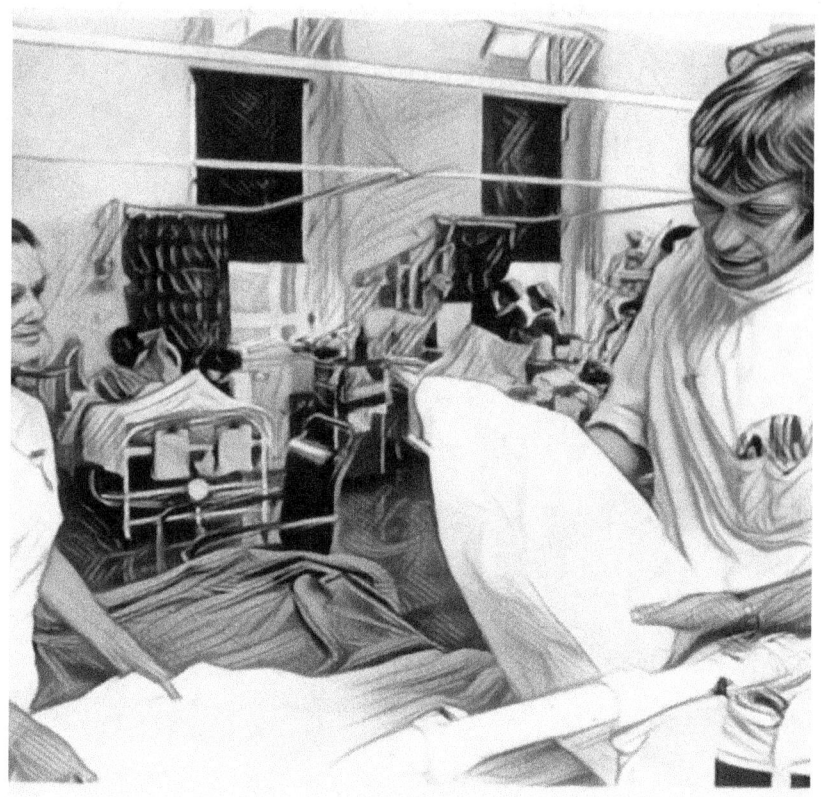

The Nightingale ward was very common during my UK nursing days though there were certainly many modern hospitals at this same time with smaller 'bays' where say 6 or 8 patients might be, as well as private rooms. The Nightingale ward was a large room subdivided with cloth curtains separating the beds and the patient in them, allowing for some privacy, however you could hear everything that was going on within the pulled curtains.

The patient's head of the bed would be up against the wall, and you could walk down the *centre* of the ward and see all the patients on your left and right with spacing between beds. You could see them at a glance.

This style stemmed from the late 19th century and was inspired by Florence Nightingale. She felt the layout and the big windows of these wards would be conducive to healing with the sunlight from the big windows and the cross ventilation as these windows could open, and this was before there was A/C.

Stateside, I worked in a hospital that had 2- 4 patient bed bays within a ward and there were private rooms, which at the beginning of my time as a US nurse, were a bit of novelty. You might need to require it medically, otherwise it was a bit of luck.

Many contemporary or recently built hospitals are now private rooms only! I worked in a hospital that had couches that were pullout beds for relatives in each room.

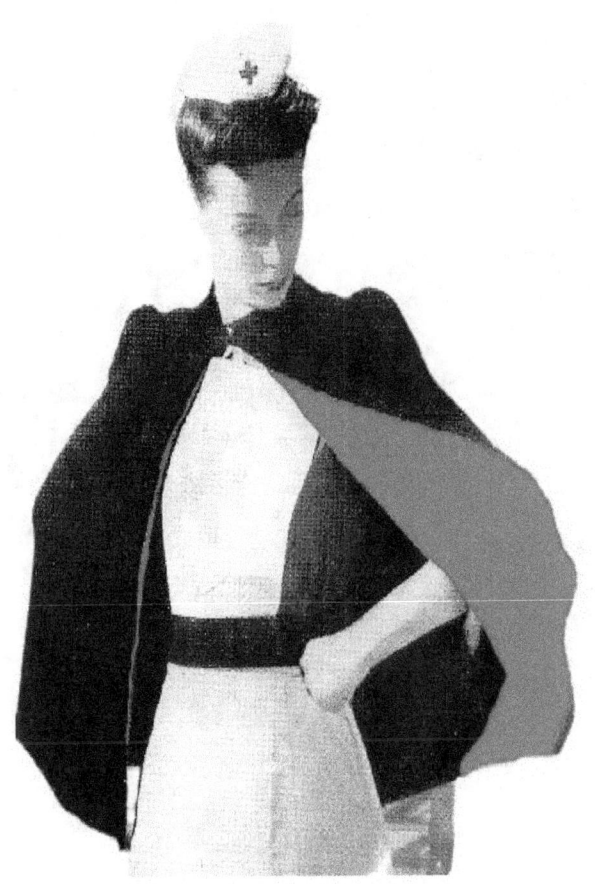

Theatre

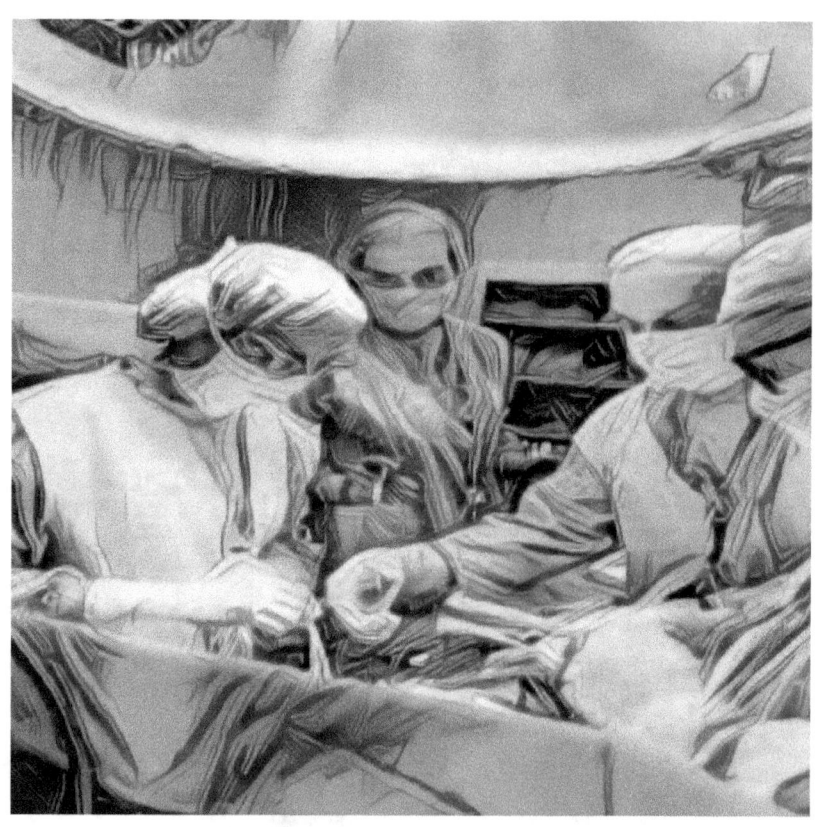

Off to theatre my boy! Yes, that's the correct spelling! A place where one went to have surgery or an operation as it was also called. Surgery is like a performance with many people involved with their very specific roles. The surgeon, the nurses, the anesthetist all coming together to work on this one patient.

Much the same as in the US, there are lots of checks and double checks to ensure correct patient and procedure. There are many disciplines involved with having everything run smoothly. I realized during my theatre experience that I had more pleasure engaging with patients that were awake and this rotation was not destined to be my endpoint, after I was done training.

White Coats

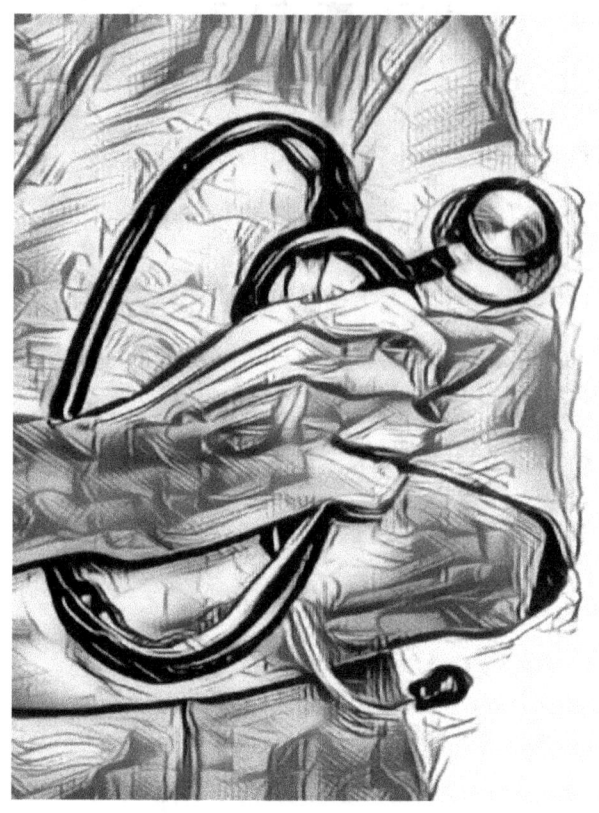

Physicians were called Doctor, when they became a consultant, they became Mister.

The younger doctors who were at the various stages of their medical training were often more personable and social, easy going and approachable.

Sometimes there were off campus out of work and training opportunities to socialize. Letting your hair down and enjoying a laugh and casual banter was always a welcome outlet from the formality and rigor of hospital life.

The relationship with MD's in the US had to be different in that we practiced in a different way. We called them to give updates on a patient's condition, reporting labs, requesting new orders as needed. Making rounds with them if called for and being called on to answer questions about a patient.

It was more likely you would know the doctor by name, how he or she specifically liked things to be done for his patient and could oftentimes develop a rapport as he or she got to know you. This would be the making of a good team that worked and collaborated together.

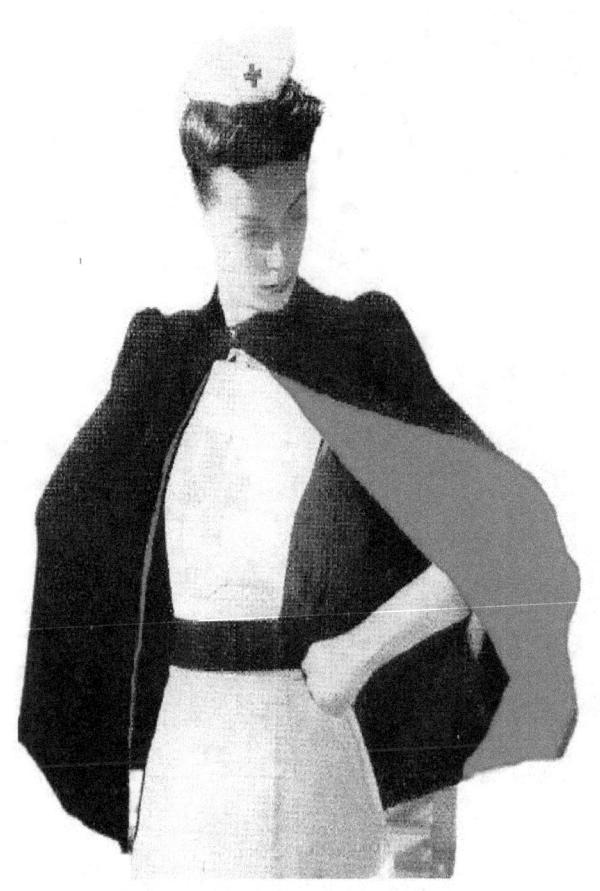

—   —

The Changing Face of Medicine

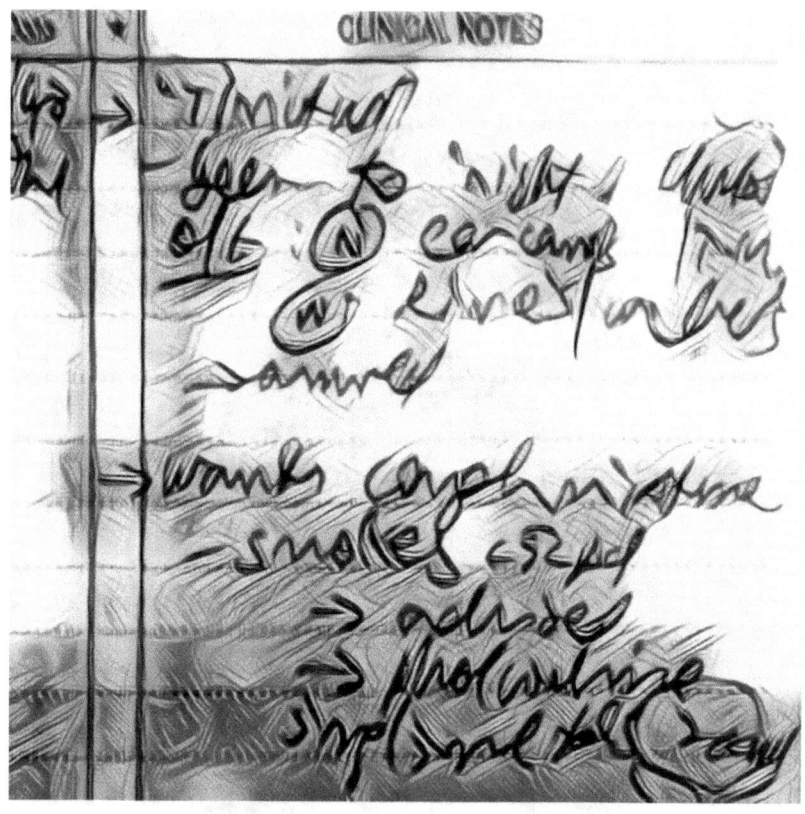

It's the pre-digital era. Doctors' orders, the direction for a patient's care were not taken verbally over the phone. Doctors would personally hand write all prescriptions or orders in person. That might mean coming into the hospital in the middle of the night if a new order needed to be made.

We have come a long way with electronic prescriptions, however back in the early days, stateside you could receive a phone order and a verbal order. You would read back for accuracy. The doctor was required to sign off by a certain time, essentially approving the instruction given.

The Essentials

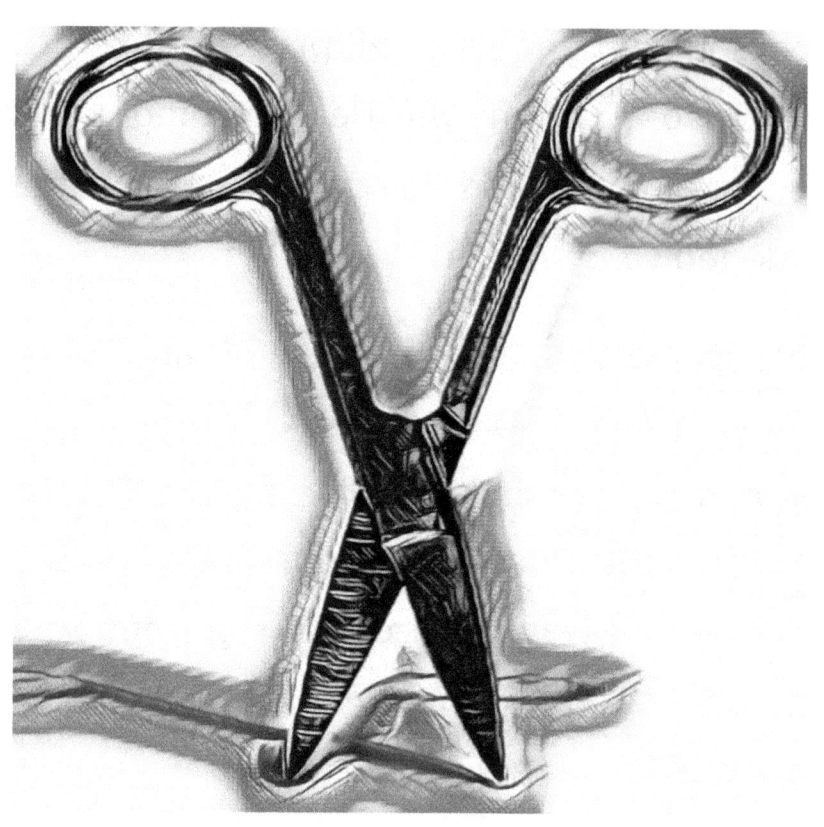

My 1st pair of nurse's scissors with the pointed ends! It was gifted to me by the staff at the nursing home I was working in temporarily while waiting to start the nursing course. This was considered an essential tool every nurse would have.

It was important for cutting tape, bandages, open packages of medical supplies and considered essential, note it was not a bandage scissor with the rounded ends. We managed to repurpose a protective cap from the IV fluid bags that would otherwise have been discarded and used that to cover the pointed end of the scissor and not injure ourselves when it was in our uniform pockets.

Imagine I still have a physical item from the age of 18. It has been packed and traveled everywhere I have lived.

I remember the day they gifted it to me; I got the feeling they were very proud of me. Going off to nursing school was considered a noble career.

I still have those scissors; today they remain sharp and shiny.

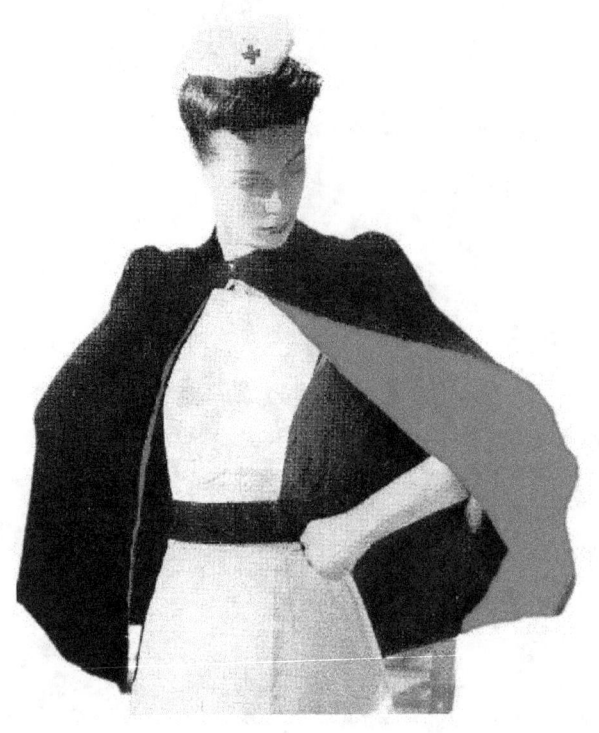

A Treat

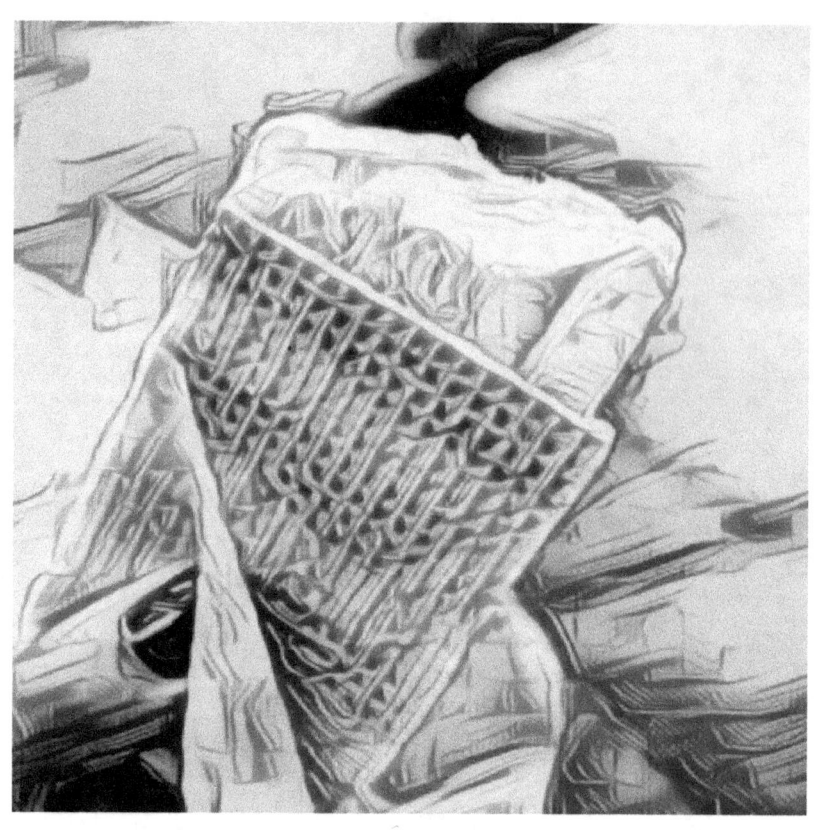

An ice cream wafer sandwich was such a delight, a treat at lunch time in the hospital cafeteria. The vanilla ice cream, and it was only vanilla, came wrapped in a plain white paper. The folds in the paper securing the ice cream were predictable and likely one would open it the same way every time, with great anticipation for that first amazing, never disappointing bite.

English ice cream , while yes I am biased, is to this day incredible ice cream. The vanilla is Creamy and delectable. It is one of my favorite things, top of my foodie delights back in the UK.

Teamwork

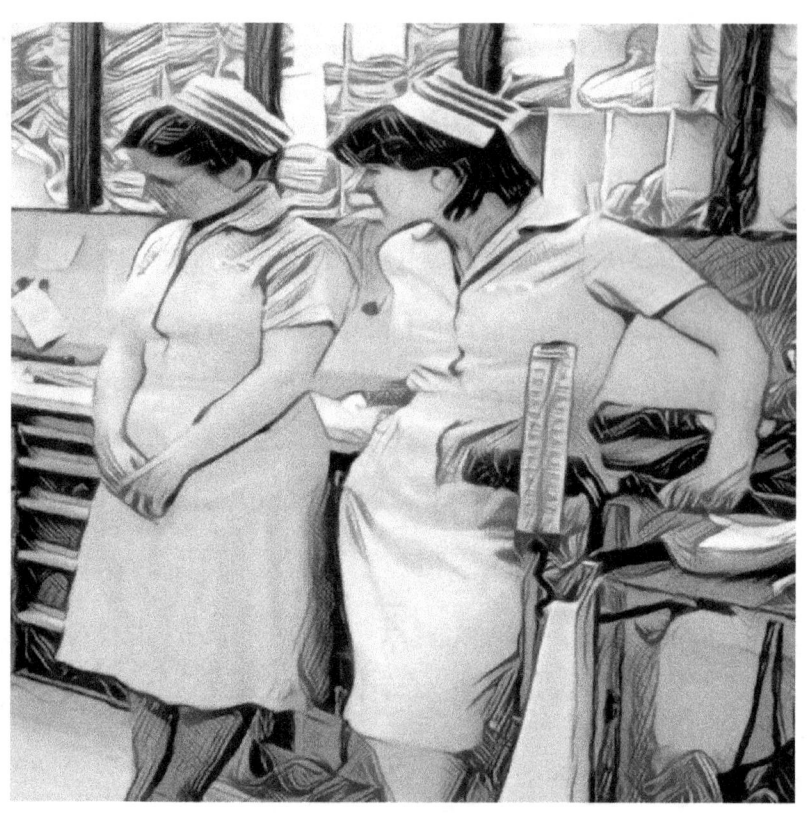

No one leaves until all the work is done! As student nurses we all worked as a team and did the bulk of the work. There would be a few staff nurses per shift, as they were fully trained and licensed. However, they were responsible for guiding teaching and the general running of the unit as well as rendering care that could only be done by licensed staff.

Just because one was done with their assignment or patients didn't mean you left. One would likely hear, go and do a 'sweep' of the unit, make sure everything was in order and support colleagues who might need help. We left together.

Depending on the 'culture' spoken and unspoken rules of the medical facility where one works, teamwork is still seen and appreciated. It adds to there being good morale when we feel supported.

Wear It Properly

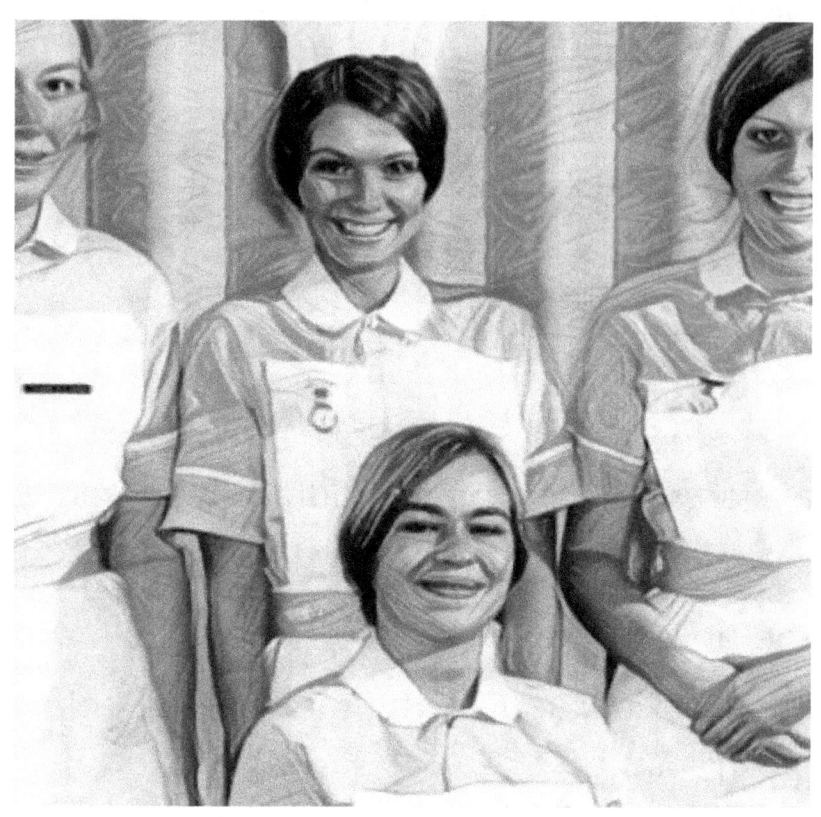

To follow the uniform guidelines meant your hair had to be off your shoulders. A fob watch was pinned to your dress. This was a wind-up watch.

The watch was placed such that you would tilt the face of the watch toward you to see the time. It would need to have a second hand for counting the pulse.

Wrist watches were not allowed and wedding bands only, a smooth metal. A ring with a stone on it was deemed unsanitary and the rough edges might scratch a patient during direct patient care.

There is still a uniform of sorts, sometimes the *colour* designated by the medical facility. In my early days stateside nurses were still wearing dresses, though not all. The requirements around accessories were much more relaxed.

Thunder

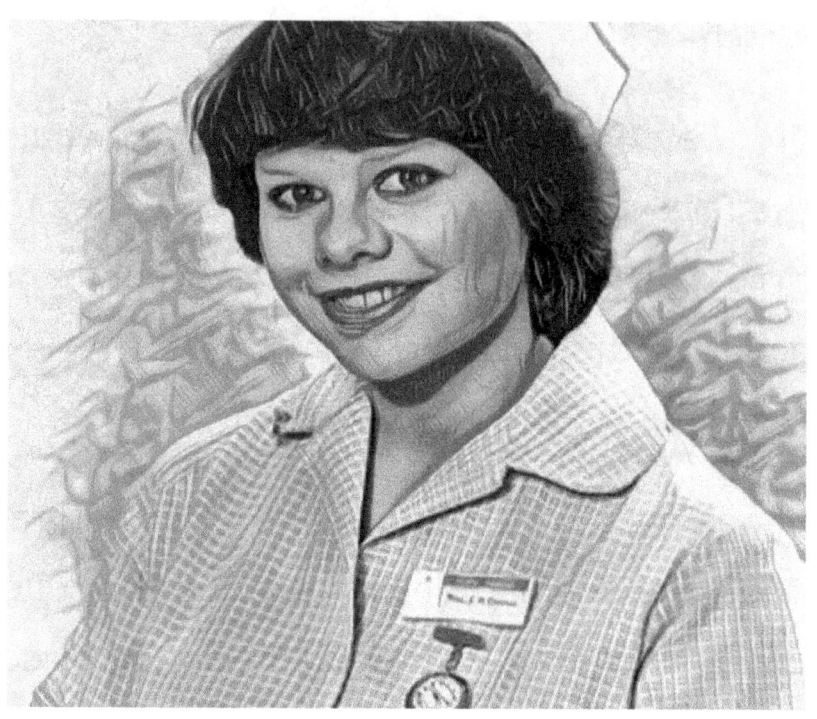

"Sometimes, nurse, when I look at you, you have a face like thunder" That was what the Sister said to me, rather spontaneously one day!

Ironically I thought of her as being rather scary. She was abrupt, and non-smiling. I didn't think she made any effort to be friendly or kind. I considered her fierce.

I didn't really see a softer side of this head nurse. She was polite and direct. I do not recall seeing her laugh or even smile.

On the evening shift at a set time, she would be brought a tray with a cup and saucer, teapot, milk and sugar and it was placed in her office for her where she took her tea break. I would often think what a nice set up that was with the cup and saucer and teapot and how I would have loved a cup of tea too!

My US experience was very different in that there was a staff kitchen where we had access to coffee that a staff member would set up each morning.

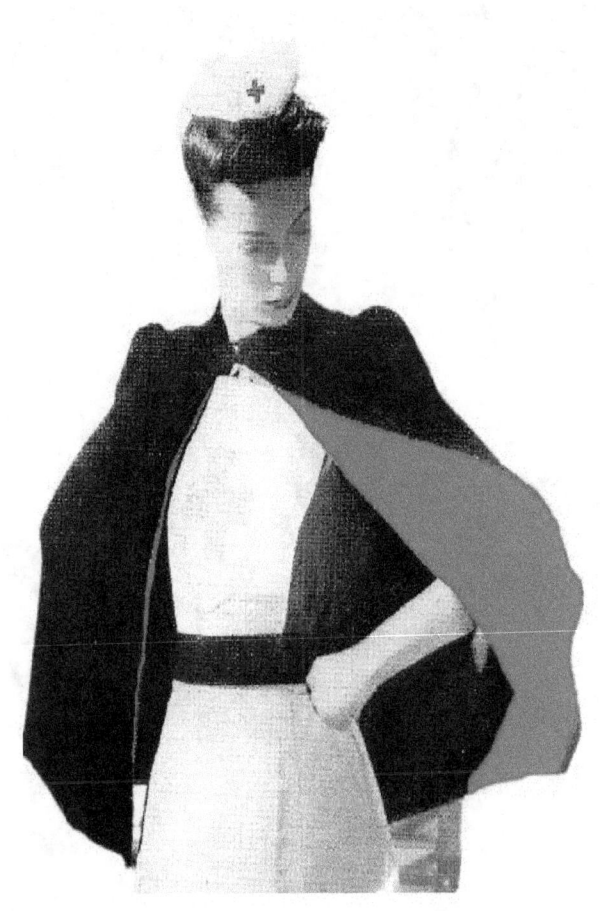

The Culture

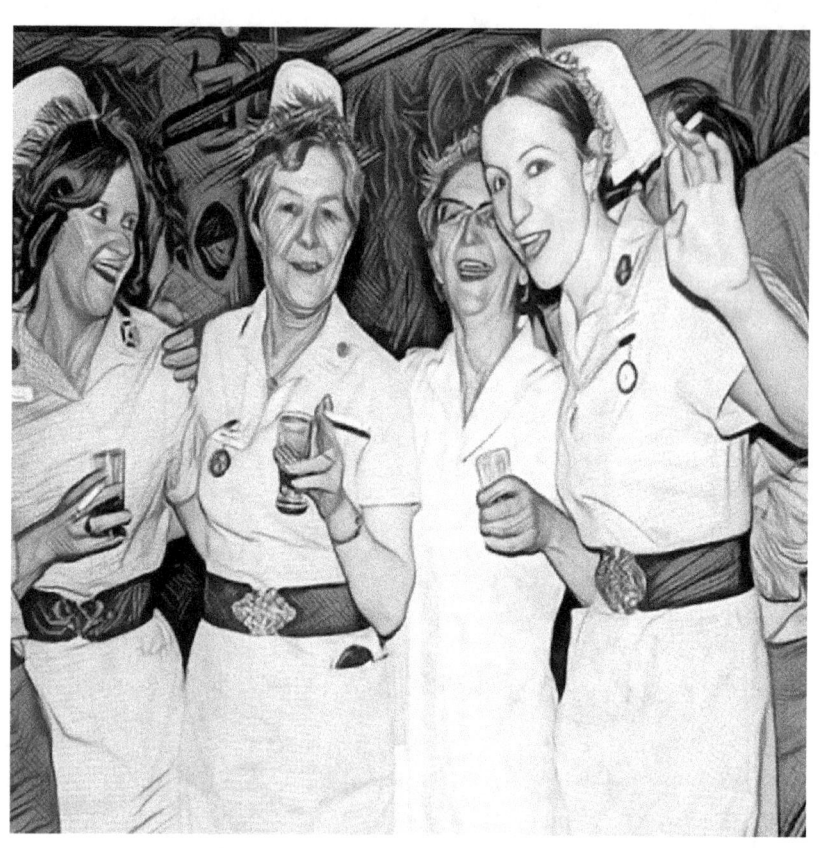

Early on in my nursing years and as a student I could return to work after lunch with the strong scent of nicotine attached to me as if I myself had been smoking. Smoking was a big part of the culture at large and nurses were no exception. At that time there weren't any ordinances about where one could smoke.

When I worked in the UK, the ban on smoking inside the hospital was not in place. However, I do not recall smoking on the nursing units in the main hospital I trained in. Possibly the nurses lounge and for the patients in private rooms. Similarly, when I came to the US, patients were permitted to smoke in private rooms.

Extended Stay

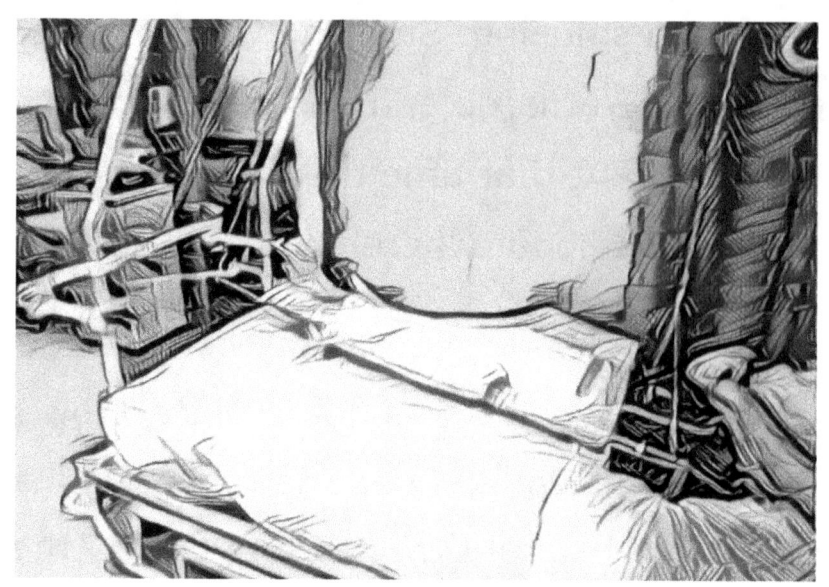

A fractured leg or hip back could land the patient in traction and hence bed rest. It was a practice used to relieve pain and keep the joint aligned and make the upcoming surgery easier. It was called skeletal traction.

Patients could be with us for many weeks, depending on the type of fracture at that time, a patient could be on bed rest in traction for 6 weeks plus.

We got to know the patients really well and they sort of became friends as well as patients.

Traction was still being used in the US when I came for quite some time.

Tea, Glorious Tea

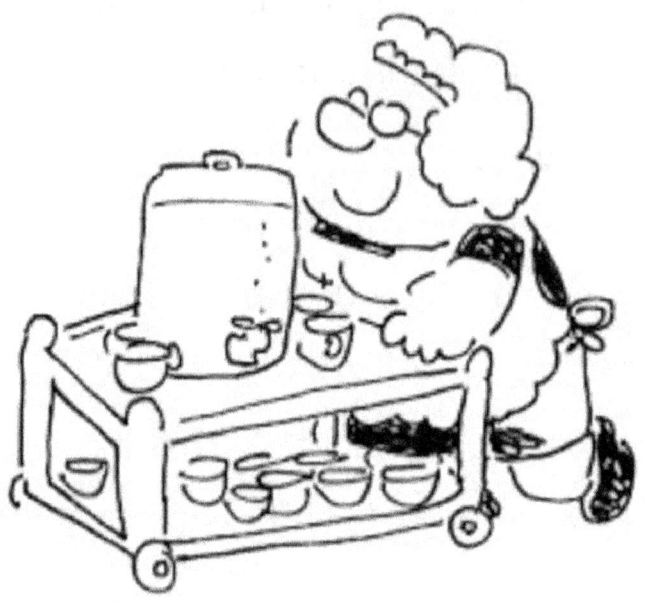

Aah, the tea round. Most sacred of rituals. Large tea bags in large teapots for those patients who didn't have a fluid restriction. Tea came with breakfast, mid-morning and midafternoon. Other times served when relatives came in for sad news such as the loss of a relative.

There were also 'sippy cups' for those who couldn't sit up enough or simply couldn't manage the cup and saucer the tea was served in.

Breakfast In Bed

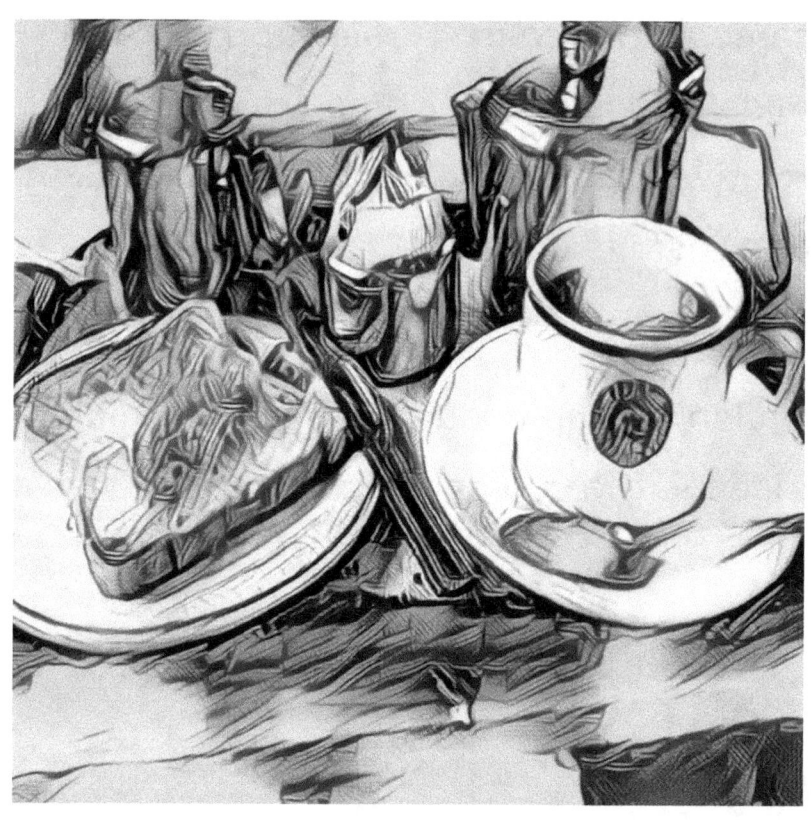

Tea and toast was considered a 'light breakfast' which was made in the kitchen that each unit or ward had access to. This is different from the main kitchen that all the meals came from. There would be a toaster and a fridge and a stove. Everything needed to make this light breakfast. This provision would be made by the student nurse or nursing assistant.

Early morning meals for breakfast prior to a procedure were provided by the food service part of the hospital in the US. The need to make tea and toast was not required anymore! I made many cups of tea not just for an individual patient but for the whole unit where I was to make a really big pot. I recall being schooled on how to make the perfect cup. Seems I needed nursing to educate me on tea making also.

Observations

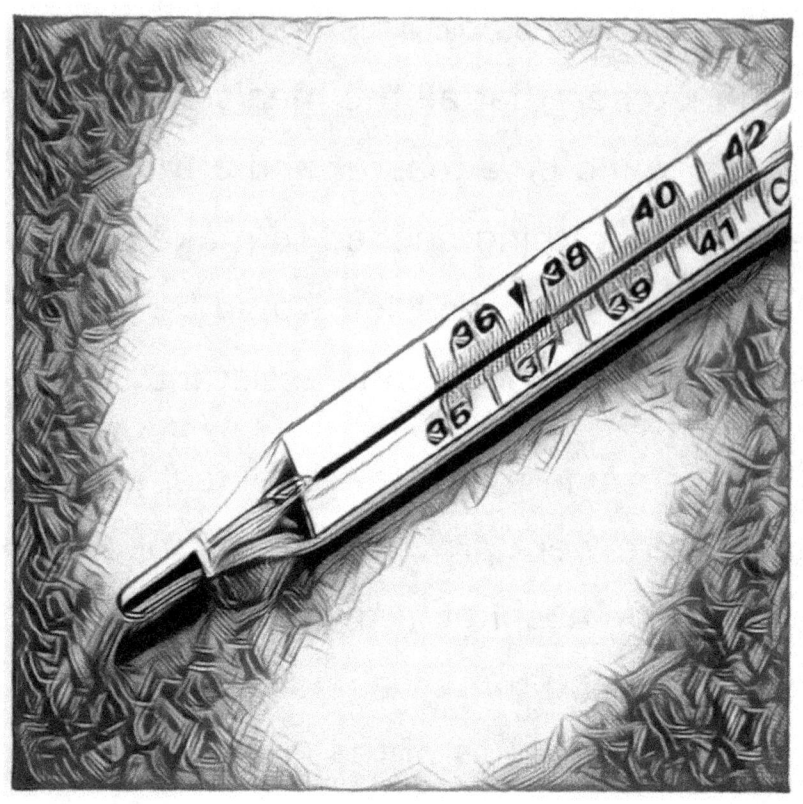

Long before they were digital, thermometers were made of glass with mercury in the middle. They were washed and reused in the appropriate cleansing solution.

There were separate ones with a red line along the glass casing, indicating this was not the one placed under the tongue, but rather 'the other end'!!

Neat and Tidy

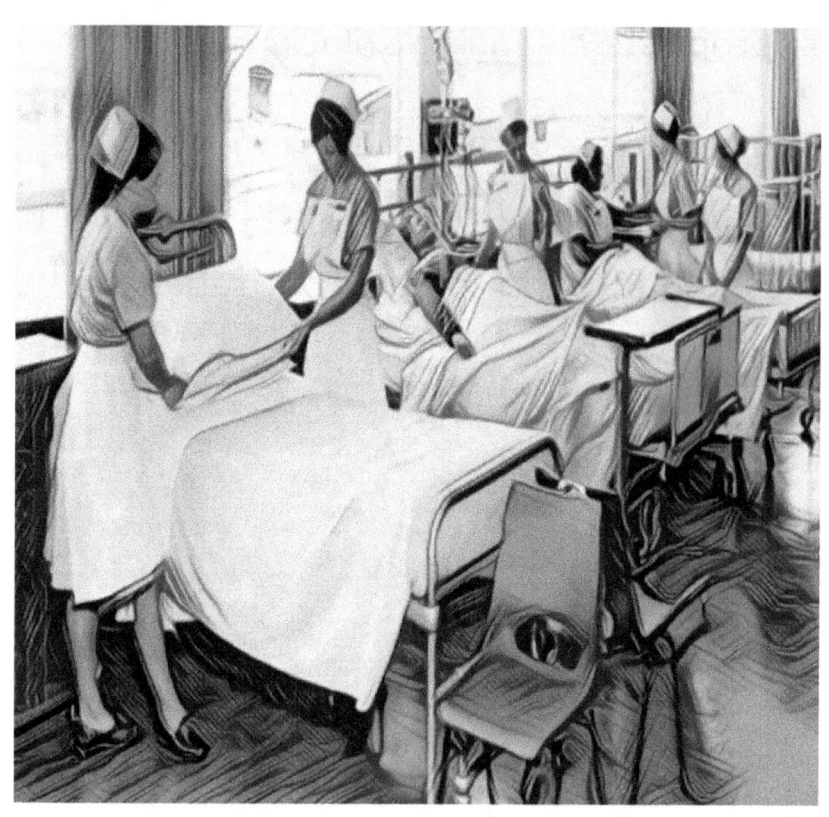

For Doctors rounds, patients and the ward needed to look and be clean and orderly. Fresh sheets for beds must be tidy and neat. The beds would be made to the standard of those times with hospital corners/folded.

The student would not address the attending consultant unless asked to do so. We knew to keep our thoughts and questions to self.

The surgical bed was a specific way of folding the sheets and blankets as if in a 'folded pack.' When the patient was brought to the bed and lifted from the trolley into the bed the sheets would not need to be pulled back but simply be opened up and the patient covered. It was a smooth synchronized process.

We did not have fitted sheets back then.

The Rules

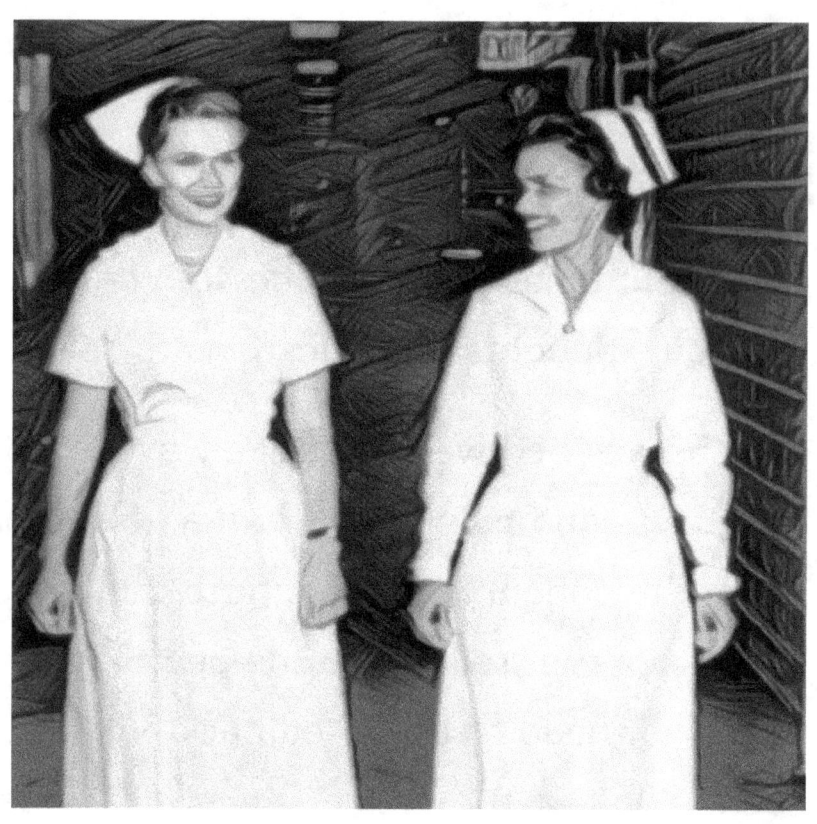

The Matron would be the modern-day version of the hospital supervisor. Overseeing all the wards or units in the hospital. She also would have a specific uniform indicating her rank.

If the nursing administrator or matron came onto your ward, you would be sure to stand up. If you happen to be wearing a cardigan as perhaps it was the night shift and a bit chilly, you would have removed your cardigan, revealing the uniform as it was intended to be worn.

The Right Shoes

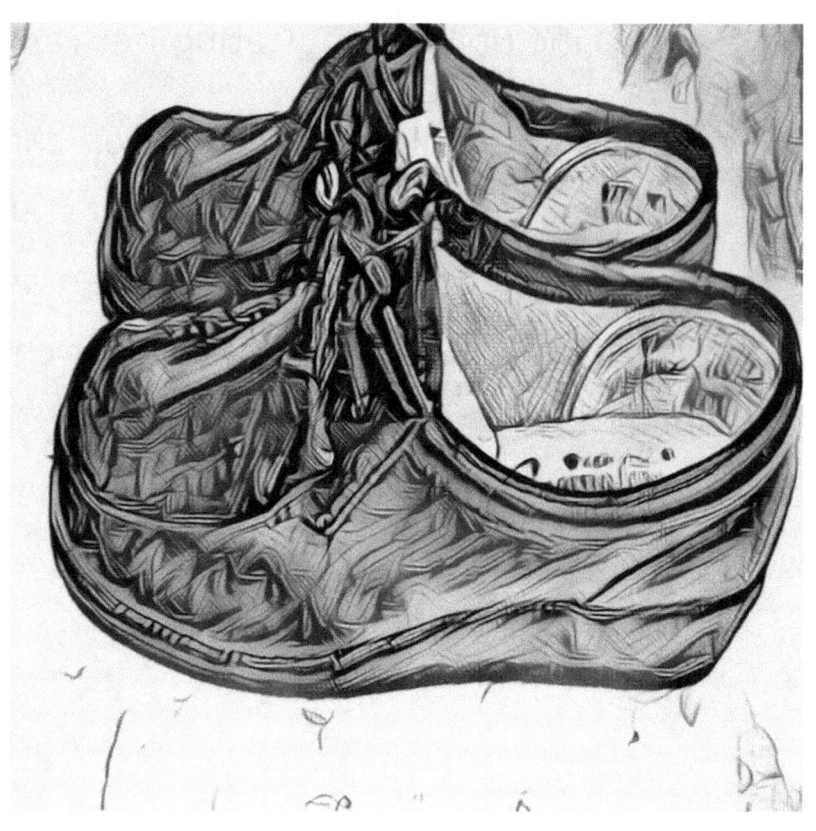

Tights as they were called (US = panty hose) were to be skin toned. The dress/uniform was a couple inches below the knee and measured by the nursing school's seamstress.

Shoes were flat, black and rubber soled.

One night while making rounds with Sister she said "nurse, has anyone ever told you your shoes are too noisy?" "No, Sister," I answered. (Well I'm telling you now, I got them changed.)

"Yes, Sister," I replied. I am still able to impersonate her Irish brogue when relaying the story to friends, though not as spot on as in years past.

Cover Up

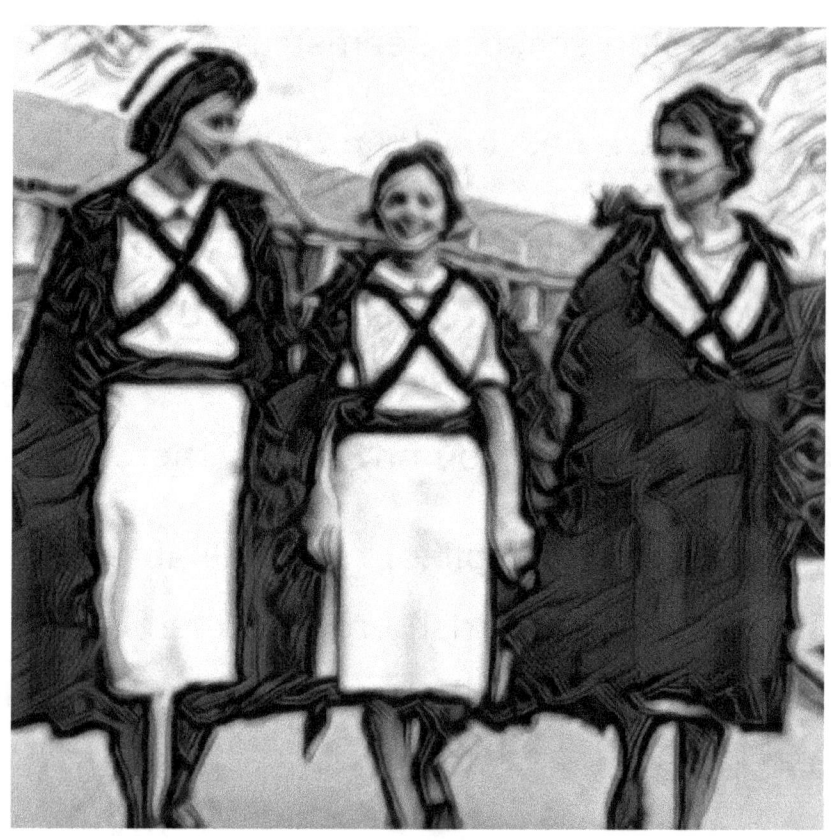

There had been a long history of wearing the nurses black wool cape! Easy to pull on around the shoulders. It covered the entire uniform, kept you warm and was to be worn on campus between housing and the wards. The nursing school also issued a button down dark coloured coat for when off site.

Often we would go from one hospital to another. Training at a different facility was sometimes part of the course.

It was considered improper to be out and about in the town and not have your uniform fully covered. That has long since changed. But those were the rules at the time.

The cape was more for being on campus between the nurses homes as they were called or dorms.
The button down dark colored 'gabardine' fabric coat was worn when in the town, city streets

when you were getting a bus to work or from one campus to another as you may have had a rotation at a different site. Most of us back then did not have a car.

This seemingly sacred practice went on the whole time I was there.

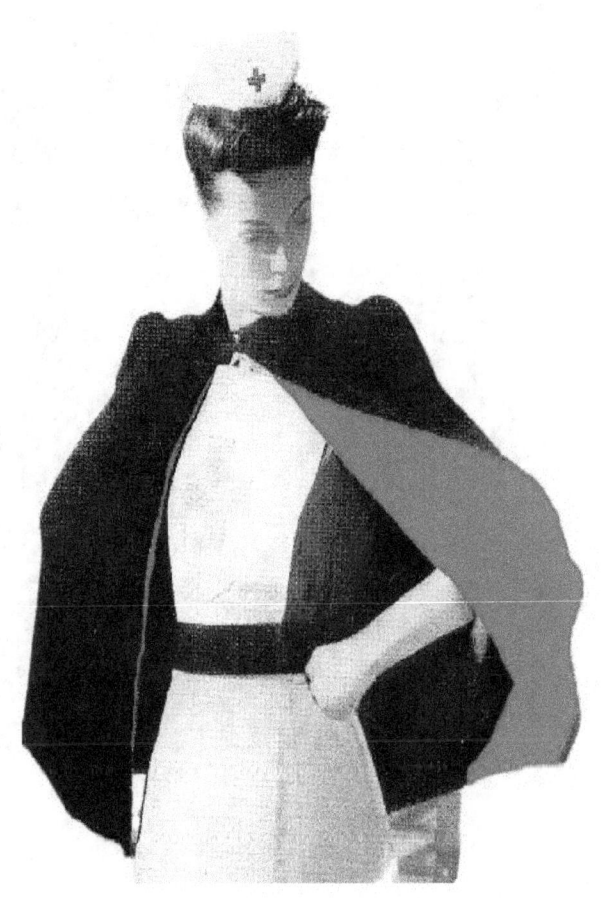

The Nurses' Home

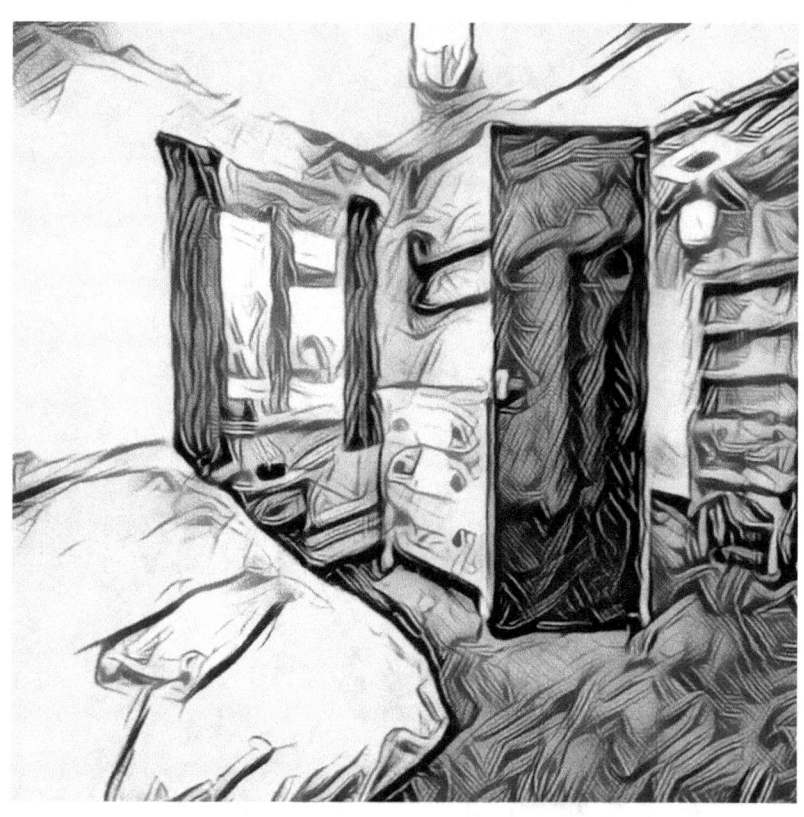

Nursing students were required to live in the 'nurses' homes' on campus. My base hospital was contemporary. It was built just a few years prior to my coming, and the nurse's home was also updated and quite comfortable. We had our own room and shared the laundry, kitchen and bathroom.

The experience in the nurses home as it was called or dorms was a good experience. I worked at what was then considered a modern hospital and the nurse's home was relatively new. We had a full kitchen where we could cook meals and a shared bathroom on each corridor for about 8 nurses. All having different shifts so it tended to not be a problem. There was a washing machine as well as a laundry service for our sheets. We were on campus so getting to class or the hospital wing when we were doing our clinical rotations was just a walk across campus. Very much appreciated after those long days.

Today's students live like other university students, they likely would be commuting to their assigned hospital for clinical experience. It was a comfortable experience with enough privacy. We would decorate our rooms to capture our personality and make it a welcoming spot, after our shift. On occasion, I had a friend come over and stay. We would spend the day having fun in the local downtown area.

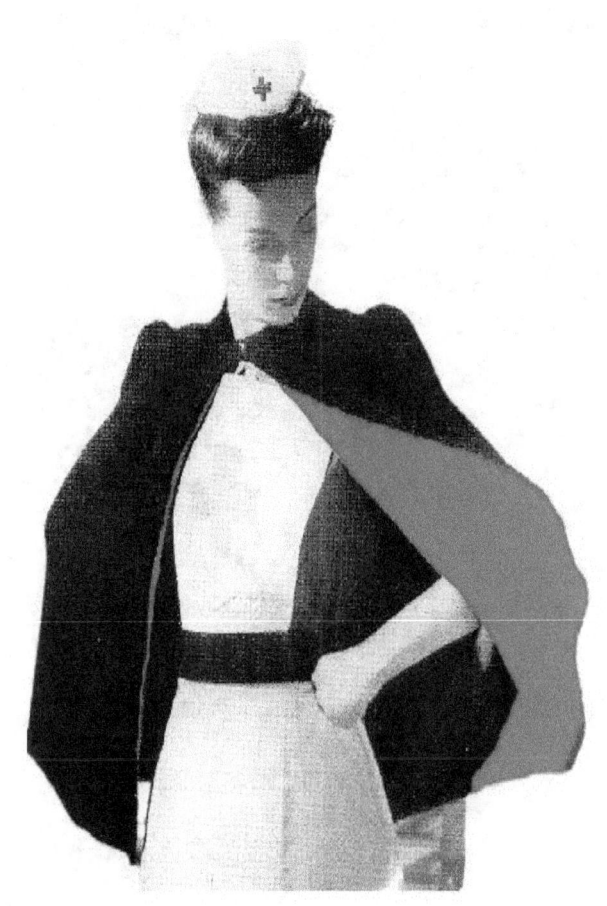

Practice-Practice

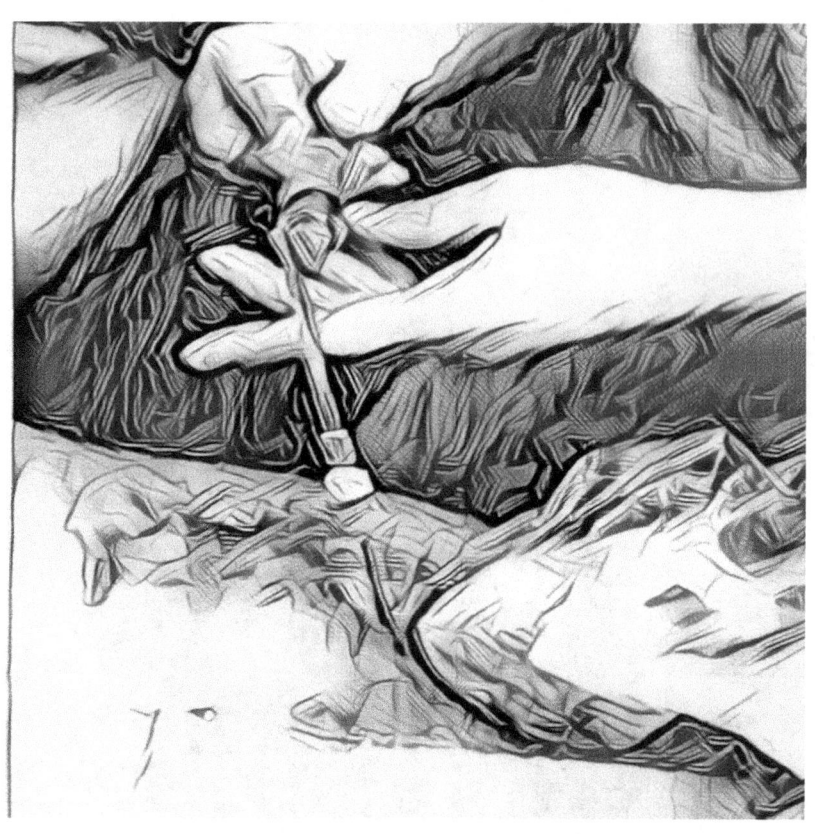

We saw so much at such a young age, most of us started at 18. We got a lot of experience. It was a teaching hospital where nurse training happened, as the hospital was affiliated with a nearby university. There were student doctors also.

I learned much and was able to participate in many procedures.

We got to witness and learn such practices as the ''Aseptic technique' which was used for sterile dressing changes where contamination of the wound incision was to be avoided at all cost and other procedures where keeping the patient free of microorganisms was of the highest importance. Any invasive procedure would require this. There was what seemed like a synchronized way to do things, it can look like an art form if watching it. I particularly enjoyed dressing changes and suture/stitches removal. It was a great skill to have.

Bedrest and Bedpans

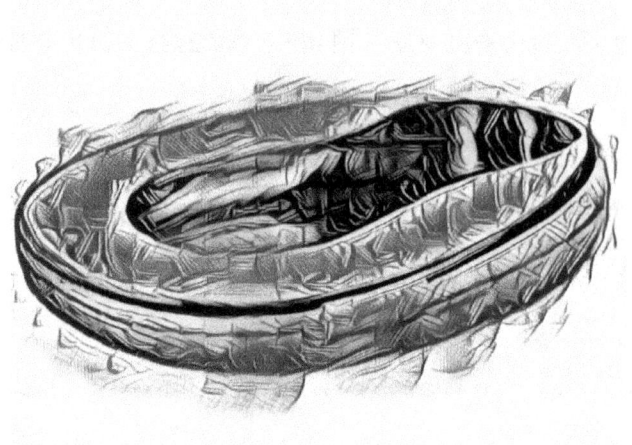

Cold hard and shiny is how I would describe these large metal bedpans for those that couldn't or shouldn't get out of bed for a host of reasons.

Over time, the bedpans began being made with some composite-type material that would be compressed in a compactor after use.

Definitely not a fun aspect of nursing life. As we help people with all aspects of daily living, going to the bathroom is one of them! Likely not so fun for the patient also. "Can you lift your bottom" would commonly be heard from behind the curtain, when passing through a nursing unit.

The Lambeth Walk

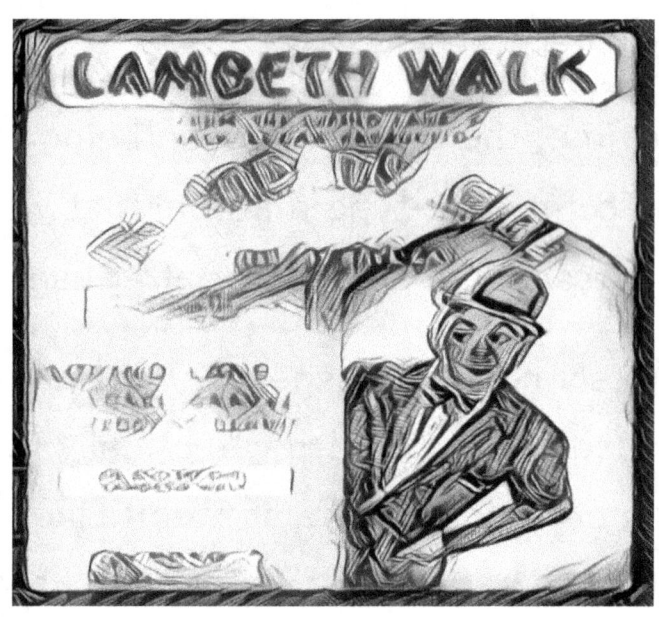

"Doing the Lambeth walk, oy!!" A song from the 1937 musical ' Me and My girl. The song takes its name from a street in London.

A fellow nurse and I sang that with a patient as we walked on either side of her, she was not strong enough to walk alone. She had some confusion related to her Parkinsonism (an umbrella term that refers to brain conditions that cause slowed movements, rigidity (stiffness) and tremors.)

It's still a fond memory, hearing her singing as we walked down that Nightingale floor.

Continental Shifts

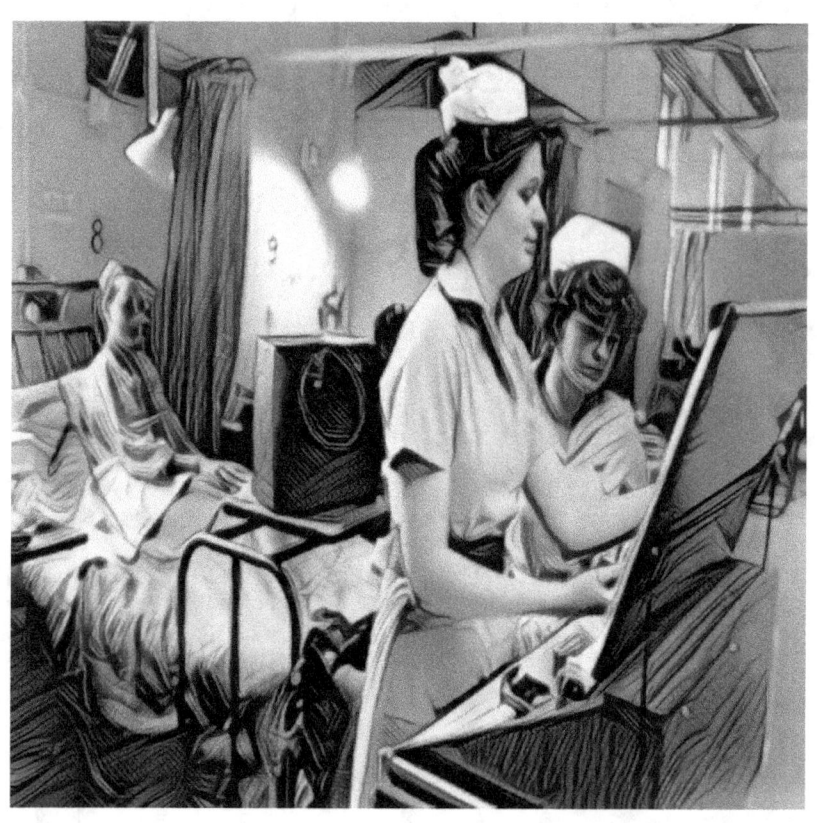

The work was hard; the hours could be extended, called 'Continental shifts.' Meaning you were not working a shift exclusively. You might be on a day shift starting in the morning, followed by an evening shift the next day, and right back to a day shift the next day after.

So, getting in from work in the evening, sometime after 9 pm, and then being on duty for the 1st shift the next day was typical.

It was very taxing at times, emotionally and physically; we, however, managed to find humor where we could and support each other.

The shift switching up from day to day was challenging, but somehow we trudged on, a bit of grumbling here and there amongst us.

In the US, you worked your selected shift only. The 'Continental Shift' (different shifts, back-toback) as they were called, happened in the

UK while we were students. Stateside, the scheduling seemed kinder, and you could plan your life accordingly.

I worked even harder in the US hospital and am convinced in those early days the hardest and fastest I had ever worked. It was amazing how intense it could be at times.

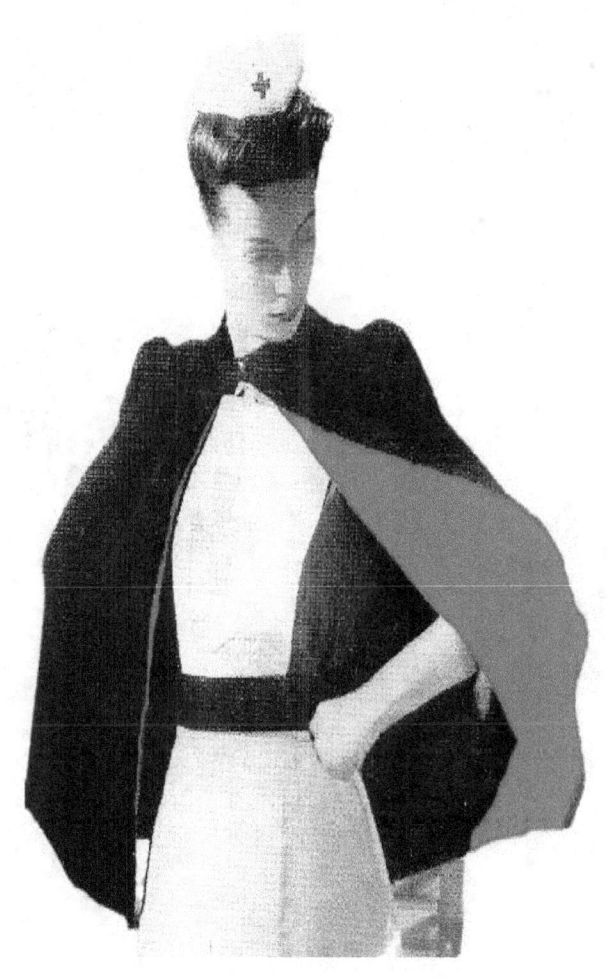

Special Touches

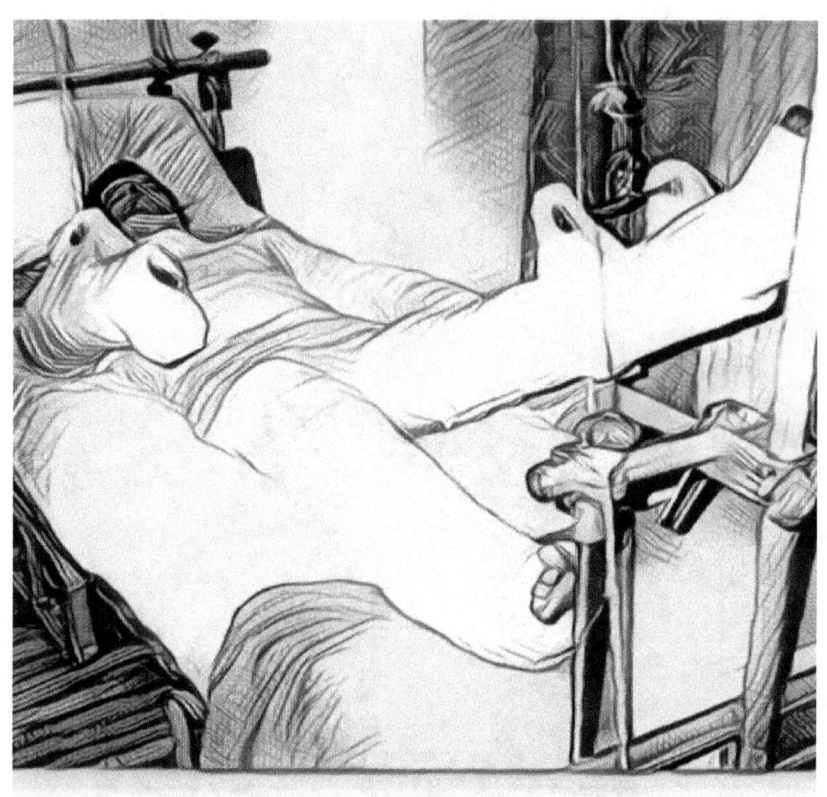

For the long stay of *orthopeadic* patients on bedrest, we were able to remove the head of the bed and wash their hair!!

We had oversized jugs that we filled with warm water and portable sinks that would be rolled up to the head of the bed and it was a team effort. Often two student nurses worked together washing the patient's hair. It was quite fun, and it made the patient feel really good.

Let Your Hair Down

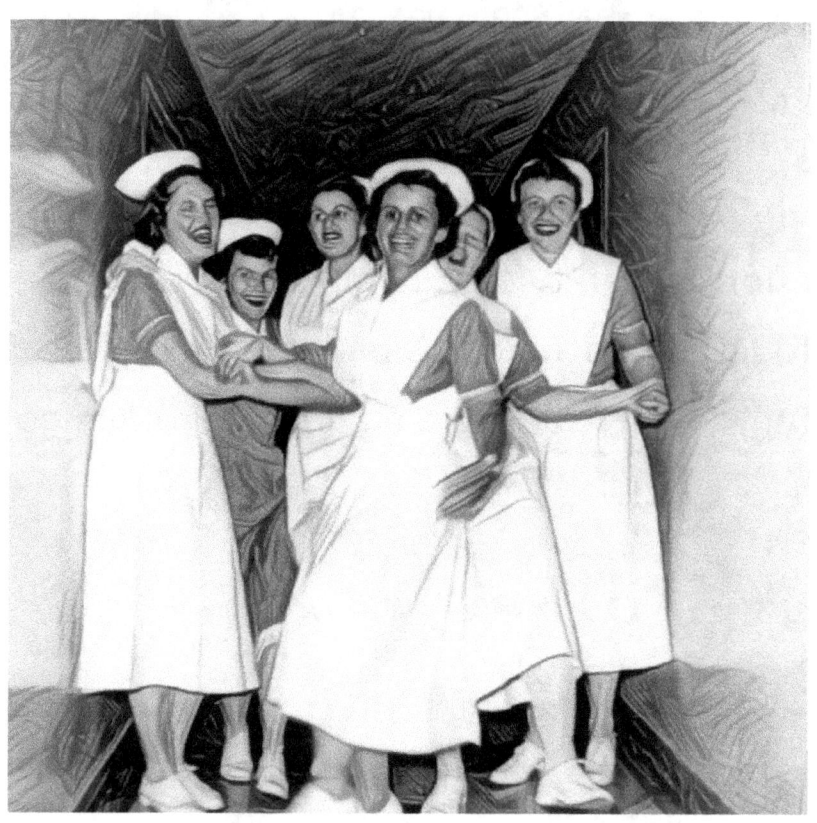

Despite the challenge of it all we nurses found a way to laugh and had each other for support. Having a good sense of *humour* was a must and finding ways to make fun of a situation helped us stay calm and carry on.

Many of us headed home to our family on occasions such as a long weekend off . We found fun, social things to do in a town, which for most of us, was not where we grew up. Dining out, shopping and for some there were parties off campus. I had a small TV in my room, as well as a record player!

Final Thoughts

Pursuing nursing as a vocation was a fitting choice due to its high esteem. I was keenly interested in anatomy and physiology and viewed myself as an educator with a compassionate nature and a quiet voice.

This book is a recollection of many instances where my peers put in a lot of hard work within a strict and inflexible structure. We were challenged at times, and yet there were rewards of being a nurse. Together we significantly impacted many lives.

Nurses are remarkable in their unwavering commitment to others, their passion, and love for the profession. Similar to any superhero, the nurse with her warm, professional cape, truly serves as protector, advocate and champion, saving lives and providing comfort even in the final moments of a patient's life. She extends her support to family members and goes above and beyond what many would do. It could mean removing her jacket and putting down her bag as she's about to leave work, already standing at the elevator, when she notices a physical therapist walking with a patient whose condition has changed and urgently asks for assistance.

At that moment, there is no one else available to help, and there is no time to search for another nurse. It becomes a collective effort to assist the patient and ensure the safety of all involved. The notion of being off duty and the patient not belonging to her doesn't apply in this case. Nurses everywhere have countless stories of doing whatever is necessary. Such events occur daily and these superheroes show up regularly on all shifts. I am grateful for my past, present, and future nursing colleagues and hope they recognize their impact on the people they serve.

www.ingramcontent.com/pod-product-compliance
Lightning Source LLC
Chambersburg PA
CBHW071215120626
46546CB00006B/2575